What Women Want In a Man

Tips to Understand what Your Girlfriend Really Wants and Build a More Lasting and Stable Relationship Over Time

Kelly Jones Lee

Table of Contents

Introduction

When I was a little girl, I would dream about the perfect man. He was the prince of a large kingdom with open fields and snow-capped mountains that reached the clouds. The kingdom smelled like cotton candy and had pink trees that lined a pathway through the forest toward the kingdom. The trees were edible, of course. Clouds could be picked from the sky and every pillow was stuffed with cloud fluff. My prince's crown was made of liquid gold and constantly shifted as he walked. His castle sat in the middle of the mountains, and the capital city's buildings had emerald and garnet roofs. The crystal roofs sparkled day and night, casting rays of rainbows over the cobblestone paths and neighboring buildings. The giant, ornate castle that I was going to live in had hundreds of rooms and a servant for every chore. The floors shone like millions of diamonds, and chandeliers were shaped like unicorns and mermaids. My prince would buy me the most lavish and extravagant ball gowns, and we'd dance every night away in the moonlight with stars shining down on us like a disco ball. Every gown would be made from different magical fabrics that shifted colors at different times of the day.

And my prince? My prince was the most dashingly handsome man in the whole world with golden, sun-kissed skin and a smile that could melt hearts. His shoulders were broad, sculpted from granite, and his chiseled chin could cut you with its sharp lines. He was tall and strong and could ride a horse without a saddle. Every maiden in the kingdom was in love with him and every girl who'd ever been mean to me was green with envy.

My dreams may have changed since then, but my dreams of the prince and the magical kingdom still make me smile. That was the first perfect man I conjured up. The first of many.

Needless to say, I never got my prince or my kingdom. I was a child with many hopes and dreams that would never become a reality. I wanted to become a ballerina princess spy with a flying unicorn as my batmobile. I wanted a talking rabbit that served me tea and a dragon that heated up the beverage with its fire whenever it got too cold. I wanted 13 children all named a different variant of 'Alice' and 'Gregory.'

As young children—and even young adults—we create these fantasy scenarios in our heads with no possibility of them ever coming true. I was never going to get a Greek god riding a unicorn bareback, but I did find a nerd who dressed up as a prince at the neighborhood fair and rode a stick with a stuffed horse head. He didn't have a castle or kingdom to look after. He didn't have fortunes a dragon could hoard, but he was real. We met an hour after I watched him rescue a damsel with a yarn wig from a tower in front of a corn dog vendor. His horse was leaning against the side of the little trailer, and he smiled the brightest smile my way. I knew then that I had found my soulmate. He might not have been a real prince with fortunes beyond compare, but he had the confidence of a prince and worked toward those fortunes.

He introduced himself as Prince Luke, dragon rider, monster slayer, and hero of damsels. Of course, he had no idea about any of my childhood fantasies. How could he? I'd never told anyone before. But that night, I realized that our perfect partner does exist. They might not come the way we expected them to, but they will show up. Many friends in the past have struggled with finding a man who ticks all their boxes. I found my prince in a cheap costume and a cardboard crown.

It was at that moment when I met him that I realized that I didn't want any of the things I'd always dreamed about. I didn't care about him being a prince, I just wanted him to have that attitude and sense of responsibility. He didn't have to be the most gorgeous being in the world, he just had to be gorgeously funny and witty. I've always wanted a man to protect me and slay the monsters that meant me harm. Luke was that person. Luke became my king, and our house became our kingdom.

I am 41 years-old with two kids, living a perfectly mundane life in a house I like to call my kingdom. I've been places, I've seen things. I've been through enough bad breakups, consoled enough friends during breakups, and set up quite a few blind dates in my time. I know what I'm talking about, and I want to make it as easy to understand as humanly possible. Sometimes I wish that my husband would pick up a damned book on how women's thoughts work and what exactly we want.

From childhood on, girls dream about the perfect man. Where boys play with cars and pretend to be dinosaurs, girls play princess and fantasize about their knight in shining armor. It puts men at a disadvantage because we had that much more time to create our perfect soul mate. We had time to create every single trait. I was that girl who used to stay up at night and dream about crowns and unicorns. The truth is that whether we know it or not, our idea of the ideal man changes over time. In my case, it matured greatly.

But there are things that most women want in men. Some things stay consistent and I, a woman who's been in many failed relationships, am here to tell you exactly what those things are and how to identify what your woman wants. Perhaps I'll spill a secret or two not even my husband knows about. You'll just have to keep reading.

Chapter 1: Nobody's Perfect

The definition of the word 'perfect' is something that is as good as it can possibly get. It's faultless and free of any defects.

Have you ever come across a person without any faults? There is always room for improvement, always some way we can be better. Everyone has a different idea of what exactly perfection is, which means there will never be a single perfect thing. No person, no object. Perfect things don't exist, and that's just how it is. Striving to be anything other than you, to be perfect in someone else's eyes, is a fool's errand. There's a reason why fictional characters are flawed most of the time. It's to make them relatable. Their flaws make them likable and, in some cases, sexy. Loki from the Marvel Universe is a perfect example. We can all agree that Loki is more than a little damaged and, in some cases, really evil. But in the end, his good exceeds his bad and his flaws actually make him a more likable character. Christian Grey is a total tool, but he's hot as heck. Why? Because he's unapologetically flawed. He's accepted it. Jon Snow is a brooding, damaged, and all around sulky male being. But that means he's a relatable character. He's emotional and will do everything for his family and friends. Jon is incredibly loyal. Forget his looks and those gorgeous locks, his loyalty despite his faults is what makes him so incredible. I can name one hundred more characters as examples, but you get the point. Fictional worlds have the ability to create perfect characters, but they don't because they want to make the characters likable and relatable. They want to appeal to women with their male characters and the creators know that the perfect man is not the way to go. We like trouble, we like damaged, and we like having something to care for and help repair. Perhaps that's why bad boys get all the girls. We like the imperfect ones.

There are certain things in life that we as humans have to know and understand to make the best of ourselves and our lives. There are things that we need to fully accept to become better and get a better understanding of us as people and what makes us who and what we are. Knowing and understanding this can benefit you and your partner immensely.

It will ease the pressure off of your shoulders. You want to be the perfect man, you want to be the man who women desire. If you didn't want to be, and if you didn't want to fully understand what goes on in a woman's head, you wouldn't have picked up this book in the first place.

My father is a difficult man. Nothing I could ever do was good enough for him. My mother always says that his flaw is expecting too much of the people around him. He is blind. He doesn't see that people aren't perfect - that people don't have it in them to be perfect. But still, my mother loves him without boundaries. She always has and always will. She accepts his flaws for what they are and focuses on the good things instead. My mother, on the other hand, talks too much. Once she starts speaking, there is no stopping her. I can see that it annoys my father, but then my mother starts babbling about art and my dad just melts. His whole body language changes and I can tell that he appreciates how passionate my mother is about art. He looks at her as if she is everything on his checklist. I guess they know that no one can be perfect, and they've accepted it.

That's what we need to do. We need to look past the imperfections or embrace them. More often than not, a woman will fall for you because of your flaws, not despite them.

Acknowledge the Facts

No one on earth is perfect. Whether it's in their own eyes or someone else's, it's impossible to be perfect. All of us are flawed in some way, and trying to deny that is a mistake. Trying to strive for perfection is a mistake you'll soon learn is impossible. But these flaws are not obstacles for you to overcome. They're a part of who we are. If you were better looking, would you have been happier? If you could get rid of your freckles, would women look at you more? If I had a firmer butt, would it stop my man from cheating? The answer to all of these questions is no. If he wants to cheat, let him cheat; it won't change the fact that I am imperfect. If only one woman looks your way, then that's the woman you want to be with.

Accepting your own flaws and imperfections is the first step to accepting your partner's flaws, instead of trying to change them. Flaws are what make us who we are as people and once we try to get rid of that, we are no longer ourselves. It takes work to realize that any form of pursuit toward perfection, whether it's your image of perfection or a woman's, is completely and utterly in vain. If love is what you are after, you have to know that perfection and love are two entirely different things. Love is unconditional and pure, whether you are perfect or not. The perfect man does not exist, and we as women understand that. We understand that no man will tick all of our boxes. It's impossible. Perhaps that is why our lists are so long. Maybe we want more options. My point is that it is useless to strive for perfection. Rather, improve on your flaws to make yourself a better version of you, because at the end of the day our imperfections make us who we are.

I was at a conference in South Africa where multiple people spoke about being perfectly imperfect. It opened my eyes to so many things, and I am grateful that I took the time to go. One of the speakers, a man a few years older than me, said something that stuck with me for years after the conference. Our imperfections make us perfect. They don't make us perfect humans, but they make us the perfect versions of ourselves. Embracing them can only lead to your own happiness. Isn't that what everyone wants? To be happy? We want to be happy so badly that we are willing to change everything about ourselves for someone who we believe will make us happy when the truth is that no one can make us as happy as we can make ourselves. Improving is a good thing; changing is bad.

Don't Fool Yourself

Don't fool yourself into thinking that there is even the slightest chance of becoming perfect without losing yourself and your mind in the process. People look perfect from the outside, but they never truly are. The faster you see and acknowledge this, the better it will be for you and your sanity. Also, don't pretend as if you are perfect, because she will see through your act sooner or later, and it will not end in your favor. The best thing you can do is be yourself unapologetically and perhaps tweak some things here and there as you grow.

There was a boy in high school that I used to be friends with. He was a weird kid and had blue hair and used to wear contact lenses to make his eyes different colors. He didn't care about authority figures one bit, but it matched his look. It matched the whole vibe he was going for with his piercings and black, painted fingernails. At that point in my life, my prince turned into a rock star and he was the closest thing I was going to get to one. The blue-haired boy was my biggest crush in high school. He had a band that wasn't very good but he was convinced that they were going places. That was enough for a teenage girl.

He caught the eye of a cheerleader. Don't ask me how that happened. She was beautiful, and I knew I could never compete with her. My friend changed his entire outlook on life for this woman. He left his friends behind to join her crew. She tossed him out soon enough, and he had no one left. The point in telling this story is that no matter how hard you try, or how drastically you change, the person you change for will toss you out sooner or later. Why? Because any person you have to change for is not the one for you. You might also lose the people who cared about you before the drastic change, too. To them, you were already your best self. I came to hate the person my friend became. I hated him for changing.

Make Sure You Know Who You Are

Take a closer look at yourself and figure out who exactly you are, what your flaws and imperfections are, what your likes and dislikes, values, interests, temperament, hobbies, goals, and strengths are. Now you ask, "But, Kelly, why is this important?" Because we are constantly growing and changing as we get older, and as we learn new things, it's important to know who you are so you don't change yourself, thinking that this is the person you are becoming. Here are some benefits of knowing who you are.

You will be happier and more content

Once you know who exactly you are, you can express yourself fully and go after what you want since you now know what that is. There is absolutely nothing stopping you from achieving your goals and getting what you want. Knowing what you want is the first step toward getting it.

The next step is embracing it. Getting what you want is what makes you happy, am I wrong?

Resistance to any form of social pressure

It's easy to cave under peer pressure, and the reason for that is that we do not always know who we are so we let other people steer us in a certain direction. Once you know who you are, you will be grounded in your values and will know when something isn't right. We so desperately want the approval of others that we are willing to become the person they want us to be. Once you know who you are, it's harder to discard those traits that make you 'you.'

Understanding others

Knowing who you are as a person is great for understanding people, as recognizing your own flaws and struggles will help you recognize those of others. This will also allow room to empathize with other people because you are aware of the things they are going through and struggling with.

Figuring Out Who You Are

There are many methods to figuring out exactly who you are, some of which might be better than those I'll be listing. Perhaps you already know who you are and you can skip this section entirely. But to those of you who still have doubts, let me tell you something. Women appreciate someone who knows who and what they are. They like men who don't make apologies for the people that they are. More than our checklists, we want a man that is real and true to himself.

Figure out your likes and dislikes

What you like and dislike is a huge part of who you are as a person. How do you describe yourself to others? "Hi, I'm Kelly Lee and I'm 41 years old. I like reading and seeing the world." Those are my likes. Take the time to imagine introducing yourself to someone and list the first things that come to mind. It's easier to identify your likes than to identify your dislikes, so start with the easiest part. When you move on to your dislikes, don't hold back. If you are unsure of something, add it to the list.

Contemplate your strengths

Your strengths and talents are as much a part of you as your nose or ears. There is nothing you can do to change that. The only thing you can do is find something you are moderately good at and work on it. If there is a challenge in your life, you might end up disliking it just because it's difficult for you to handle, do, or understand. Those are your weaknesses, not dislikes, and that can always be worked on and improved.

Find comfort

What brings you comfort in life? Knowing this tells you a lot about yourself. Is it a book? Is it your home? Is it your dog? There are many different things that brings us comfort in life. In my case, I find comfort in music. Now, you can already tell that I am a music lover.

Probe a little deeper

There's more to you than meets the eye, and no one is going to do the job of delving a little deeper if you do not do it yourself. There are hidden parts in all of us, and it's our job to find them by digging a little further than you've ever dug before. Dig out those childhood bullies, dig out the rejection to the prom. That kid is who you are. So what if they couldn't appreciate you? There is someone out there who will.

Ask yourself these questions

Here is a list of questions you need to ask yourself when discovering who you are.

- What are your interests?

- What are your values?

- What is your temperament?

- What hobbies would you like to do and which do you partake in?

- What would you do if money was not an issue?

- What do you do when you are alone and away from the influence of others?

Make a list of things you want to achieve in life

Think of it as a bucket list. What are the things you want to achieve before you die? Where do you want to be in five years, or even ten? How do you plan on getting there? All of this says a lot about your character. Do you want children? Do you want to be a proud dog dad? Where do you see yourself living? Can you see yourself settling down with a woman?

How Does Any of This Benefit You?

Knowing who you are and understanding that no one is perfect is important because it will make you think twice about changing who you are for a woman. Both sexes have a tendency to do this to get the person they believe is perfect for them. Forgetting who they are is not the correct term to use, because most of them never knew who they were to begin with. It takes a lot of soul-searching and work to find yourself, but once you have it, don't throw it away for an illusion of perfection. No one is perfect, and that is what you need to remember. No one is perfect enough to change your entire persona for. No one is worth losing yourself to. Things can be improved on or learned, but don't throw away the things you already know and possess.

Just Because No One's Perfect Doesn't Mean No One is Perfect For You

I've spent a lot of time drilling the deception of perfection into your head and what to look out for. However, just because no one is perfect, that doesn't mean there won't be a person who's perfect for you. There are things you might want in a woman that this person will not possess, and vice versa. This doesn't mean they aren't perfect for you. Don't look at the things she doesn't possess, but instead look at the things that she does have.

Everybody's Different

When we are born, we are basically a blank canvas for the world to paint. We grow up with different parents in different homes with different rules and different relationships. We are influenced by our parents and the culture we grow up in. I, for one, have a huge liking for Bon Jovi. Even as a child, I used to love them to bits. The new-aged music just sounds like noise to me and every song has the exact same beat. It frustrates me to another level. But my kids love it. They hate my music and they love this new-aged junk. I blame their father for watching too much MTV.

Everyone is different in their own special way. The tiniest thing in our life can make a huge difference in who we are. This is how we become unique individuals.

Chapter 2: Change What You Do, Not Who You Are

Most of what women want in a man can be learned and is an improvement on you as a person. These things won't change you, but instead will make you a better version of you. Sure, you're charming and funny, but adding confidence into the mix? It doesn't change who you are completely, but rather changes the way you do things.

When Luke and I first started dating, I tried my best to hide the person I was. I knew that Luke wanted a confident, self-assured, and placid woman. I was none of those things. I wasn't confident and had little to no self-assurance, and instead of being placid, I was a loose cannon. I was truly a spitfire. I still am. I didn't want Luke to know this. Luke was tall and handsome with a good sense of style and humor. To me, he was perfect. Until one day, when I couldn't take it anymore and the guilt of lying to him about who I truly was nearly ate me alive, I told him. With a laugh and a shake of his head, he had his own confession to make. One of his friends' wives was a personal stylist and would give him tips on his wardrobe. I seems so silly, but a person's style says so much about them. He no longer wore Levis and boots, but instead replaced it with suits he couldn't really afford and ties that all looked the same. When I told him about my wild side, it felt as if a weight had been lifted off my shoulders that I didn't even know was pushing me down.

This did teach us some things, though. I learned how to keep my emotions in check and Luke learned what socks to wear with brown shoes. In the end, it all worked out. But the only reason it worked out is because we confessed our lies. We both felt a little cheated that the other person lied about it, but we couldn't be too angry because we were both guilty. We were both guilty of lying about who we were, not to mention the negative effects it was going to have if we continued with it. The constant stress of the other one finding out, the tiring act of putting up our masks, even if it for something that seems so little, can have a negative effect on a person.

What is the Difference Between Improving and Changing?

A lot of people might say that there is no difference at all, and I am here to tell you that those people are wrong. There is a massive difference. In fact, they are two different things entirely. Improving means that you are using what you have a foundation to build on, whereas change throws that foundation out entirely and starts fresh. Change is good in many ways; moving furniture around, moving houses, getting a new job, but it is not good when you are focused on your own person.

Change is doing something that is completely different, that makes you a different person, whereas improvement makes you better at being who and what you already are.

The accusation stings when a person says, "You've changed." Why? Because it's a bad thing. People don't want you to change because you are you and that is why they love you. They didn't start hanging out with the changed version of you. They started hanging out with the real version of you, thinking that you would never change, just become better. No one ever threw an insult saying, "You've improved," because it's a good thing. You need to learn the difference between the two.

Why Should I Improve Myself?

Each day, we grow. With each book we read or write, we get better. With every painting, we learn more about colors. With every meal we make, we learn something new about spices. Everything we do in life teaches us new things. Why can't we improve our personalities in the same way, too? Think of it as skill-building. But where you improve your skills for work, instead you improve your personality and bad habits. It's important to keep growing as the world grows. If you stay the same 13-year-old boy, you won't ever get anywhere because you won't be learning and growing. Women love men who work on themselves, who try to be a better version of themselves and never stop growing. It's one of the things I love most about Luke; his spirit whenever he has to tackle something new, whenever there's a challenge in front of him and he knows he'll have to improve to conquer it. Think of learning about what women want as an obstacle, and by improving yourself, you can overcome the roadblocks.

Ways to Improve Yourself

Read

Never stop reading. Whether it's fiction or self-help, reading teaches a person a lot. You can learn a lot from a well-written character. I make a point of reading to my kids every night before bed. Fiction stories, of course. Fictional characters are created to be likable and people should strive for that. Find the similarities between you and those characters and see where you can improve on your own traits.

Self-help books are just as handy even though I find them tedious and sometimes filled with a bunch of nonsense that I am never going to use. That is why I wrote this book. Find the books that will actually help you and learn from them. There's nothing as satisfying as finishing a book knowing that you've learned something or know how to improve your own life and understanding.

Pick up a new hobby

So, you've found out that this woman you're interested in enjoys rock climbing. What now? Well, my friend, swallow that fear of heights and get climbing. Trying it out won't hurt you, and you might just find something you like and are good at. Be open to trying a hobby.

It's a bonus that women love men who try new things and aren't afraid of a challenge or two, it's important to them to know that they shouldn't be scared to suggest doing something new. It helps you and your relationship, so this is definitely an important step to follow.

Overcome your fears

Whatever your fears are, they are not going to score you any points with the ladies. Many men have a fear of approaching and talking to women, but we appreciate a man who can walk up to us and start a conversation. Women are not likely to make the first move. It's not how some of us are wired, so it's up to you to swallow the fear and approach us. We feel the same way about approaching other things that scare you.

Step out of your comfort zone

Much like getting a new hobby, stepping out of your comfort zone is a great way of improving yourself. Talk to new people at a club you've never gone to before. You might just meet someone interesting in the process and pick up a new interest.

Ask a friend

Jenna, my sister in law, is brutally honest. She is so honest that she sometimes comes across as rude. Not many people like her, but I like her for that exact reason. Whenever I am unsure about something or need advice, Jenna is there to push me in the right direction. She doesn't sugar coat things. That's the friend you want to go to for this tip. Go to that friend you're usually afraid of asking, and ask then what you can improve on as a person. Trust me, I've asked Jenna and she didn't hold back. Sometimes we are blind to our own faults and traits and we need someone to help us see that.

Let go of the past

Sometimes we linger in the bad shadows of the past. This holds us back. Letting go of that prom date that stood you up will help you get rid of the fear of asking a woman out. You don't think it's still there, but it is, buried deep, deep down. Letting go of it will help you immensely.

Go on dates

Dating will give you a lot of self-confidence. Whether you are new to the dating scene or just getting back into it, don't be afraid of going out for a few drinks or dinner with a woman. It'll make you comfortable with the fairer sex. Women adore a man who can talk without babbling.

Chapter 3: Parents Have an Influence, Too

When I was four or five years old, I used to organize a wedding in our backyard. I had my grandma bake us cookies, picked flowers from the neighbor's garden because I wasn't allowed to pick ours anymore, wrapped myself in a white sheet, and waited for my father to come home from work so we could get married. My father has always been a role model to my brother and I even though he was hard on us both. We knew he only ever wanted the best for us and our futures. He was the strongest and tallest man I knew and I wanted to marry a person just like him when I grew up. Little did I know back then that our relationship was going to get rocky with me growing in age and getting sick of his constant judgment. Still, at that age, I knew nothing other than my father was a superhero. I remember the weddings as if they happened yesterday. My brother was the preacher who married us and my mother played the piano when we entered the living room for the reception.

Like most girls, my father was my hero and without knowing it, I wanted a man just like him. There as no man that worked as hard as he did, and no man who could build things as good as he could. I found myself wanting a man who could do all of those things, a man that was committed to his job and was proud to do it. I wanted a man who could build me a bookcase because my father could. A lot of women look for their fathers in men and it's not necessarily a bad thing. They know that you are not their father, they just want that same sense of security they felt whenever they were around their fathers. I also wanted a man who would raise our kids as well as my father did and marry them beneath the maple tree in the backyard every Friday. I did marry a version of my father, but let's say Luke is a little different than my father. Luke doesn't judge or preach, which is something I've grown to hate about my father. For that, Luke had other negative things like never taking his plate to the sink, but that I can handle. Luke makes me feel safe and protected, he builds whatever I ask him to, and he is ambitious and successful. Those were things I wanted to marry as a child when I looked at my father.

But why do we do this, exactly? I went and did my research because my curiosity was piqued when I realized I basically married my father.

In a perfect childhood, fathers are always there. They always have a soft spot for their little girls and they tend to spoil and care for them more than necessary. At least, that was what the research told me.

Fathers shape our perceptions of what we can expect in a man and what we should look for, or what's acceptable in a partner. Our close relationships with our fathers mean that we can make better choices in our love lives as well.

There is a difference between women who grew up without fathers and those who were privileged enough to have ones.

Women who had fathers growing up are not desperate for male companionship and approval. We can wait until a man like our father comes along. We usually have a very set checklist that we are looking for because we associate the security we felt as kids with our fathers. Some women, however, go for the complete opposite because they want to get away from their fathers. This usually happens when a woman wants to have a better and more stable relationship than her mother had and that she experienced as a child.

Women who grew up without fathers tend to seek any form of male approval, making terrible mistakes on their mission to find a person to replace the father they never had. They weren't cared for in the same way as I was and are willing to date trash in order to get it.

Of course, all of this is purely stereotypical and this is my first book, so what do I know, right?

Just like fathers, mothers also have a terrible tendency to influence a women's taste in men. Depending on how much her mother complains about her father or the things that are wrong in her life, a woman might want to avoid it altogether and take her mother's advice.

When we are children and we look at our parents as we grow up, we learn what we want in a relationship and what we don't. If your parents fight all the time, you will know that it's not what you want and you will look for something else. Perhaps it is all you know, and you believe that it is normal. The truth is that everyone takes in and processes information differently and how our parents are also affects everyone differently. It's just one of the things that makes people so unique.

The thing to remember is that women might think they want to marry their fathers without knowing that there is anything better out there. They want to marry the people they grew up with and in some cases, it's up to you to change her mind. Don't turn into her father. Show her that there is something better out there. It might be normal to her and she doesn't know that anything else is acceptable or even out there. It's the same with men and their mothers.

Another thing to consider is what she was taught growing up with her parents. What did her parents tell her to look out for, to be careful of, to avoid, and what is good?

Parents just want the best for their children and their approval means a lot to a woman. The influence parents have on relationships and the sort of person you end up with is ridiculous. Some people fight against it while others let their parents dictate the entire relationship. Luke's mother has never and probably never will approve of me, but it doesn't matter to Luke. He is one of the people who don't care. But it was very important to me for my parents to approve of Luke, especially my father. Now it feels as if Luke and my father are in a relationship instead of me.

We don't always realize how big an influence our families have on what we look for in men and what we don't.

For example, I have this uncle that drives me completely mad.

I was 12 and my cousin was 13 when I went over to their house to swim. I used to spend most of my time there, as they had a pool and we didn't. On that day, I realized why I could never stand him.

My brother and I were both in the pool with our two cousins. I can't remember what we were playing, but I remember that it was so much fun, we didn't want to leave. After a while, our parents joined us and the kids got on the shoulders of the adults and we had to wrestle for victory. The victors got an extra scoop of ice cream. My mom and I beat both my uncle and aunt, along with my brother and dad. Everyone was a sport about it, even congratulated us with handshakes just like they did on TV. All except my uncle, who accused us of cheating and moped on the side of the pool until it was time for ice cream. I didn't care much. It didn't bother me that he was a bad loser. I was used to playing monopoly with my brother. I could handle a man who couldn't stand losing.

But when my aunt built our ice cream cones, my mother and I getting our extra victory scoop, I walked out the door to rejoin my cousins and brother, I got tripped and my ice cream fell from my hands. True as Bob, there my uncle stood, leg stretched out with a stupid grin on his face. He shouted at me for dropping it and I wasn't allowed to get any more ice cream because I was "too clumsy." No one believed that an adult tripped a child so I was grounded for lying, too. That day, I swore never to date a bad loser or a liar. I knew what to look out for.

The reason I told this story is because most women had experienced in the past that completely put them off of certain traits. That also influences what they like and don't. Everything that could have taught them something, did. And that is why some women are so very picky.

It's Not Always Your Woman Speaking, it Might be Her Parents

Sometimes, more often than not, parents enjoy interfering with their children's relationships and it can go south very fast. Women want both their parents and partners to be happy, and that can sometimes lead to arguments and misunderstandings. Remember that these are the people that raised her. They made her who she is. These are the people that taught her everything she knows. She's not likely to take the side of the man she only recently met. A woman wants a man who can handle her family and not force her into choosing between the two. That's just a thing only a jerk would do.

A lot of times during an argument, whatever her parents said will be coming through. If her parents don't like you, they might be spiteful and feed her thoughts with doubts and ammunition against you. They are her parents, so why would they lie to her, right? They just want her to be happy. The key to this is not to take it too personally and to handle it calmly. Don't go accusing her parents of being wrong, and don't tell her she's being an idiot for believing them. Take a deep breath and tell your side of the story calmly if it even gets that far. Change her mind with actions, not words. Talk is cheap, after all.

The same goes for the image they sent in her mind for a man. Make her see that their idea of a perfect man for her isn't the only option out there. If she still doesn't bite, get out of there, friend. You'll be dating her family instead of her and it will just get worse when you marry her. She is not the one for you if she chooses her family over you when they are being unreasonable. Take it from someone with experience.

Chapter 4: Just Because She Has an Image in Her Head Doesn't Mean You Have to be That Man

Let's talk about expectations versus reality, shall we?

You know when those fast food joints advertise a really good-looking burger but when you get it it's as big as your palm and tastes as plastic as a Lego? Sometimes we think we want something but when we get it, it's not at all the way we expected it to be. That's the same with women. Women often have this idea of a man in their heads and when they finally get that man, they are wildly disappointed because that's not what they dreamed of at all. So, she wanted a rich entrepreneur with seven cars and a butler, but what she really got was a pompous idiot with a big head and too much money for his own good. So, just because we want something, that doesn't mean it's what we really had in mind.

It's possible that, when someone completely different crosses her path, she can fall hopelessly and madly in love with him instead of her Christian Grey. Just because she wants something does not mean she is going to be happy about it when she gets it, and she might just need someone different to make her see that she's been delusional all this time.

I am going to get killed for telling this story, but it fits so perfectly, I can't help myself.

Holly and I graduated the same year. At the time, I was still with my high school sweetheart Ben and Holly didn't have anyone. She was always holding out for this one person, this one perfect man that was going to be her one and only. She didn't see herself dating a lot of men to get to the good one. Oh no, she wanted the first one to be absolutely perfect. I never had the heart to tell her that wasn't how it worked. I couldn't tell her that taking the first, best man that checked the list was a bad idea. You had to date a few guys, go on some dates and hang out before you lose yourself. You had to know what to look out for, to learn what you wanted and what you didn't like. A relationship isn't something you can just get right the first time around. If you do, you're very lucky but most of the time, that doesn't happen.

In college, Holly met Sebastian. Oh, he was a gorgeous man, and all the ladies swooned when he passed. Holly instantly lost her heart and I knew that trouble was coming. I could feel it.

Sebastian was everything she wanted in a man. His family was filthy rich, and he had a fancy car. He was a quarterback but was smart, too. He was too smart. The man made Holly laugh unlike anyone I had ever seen before, and I would catch her dreamily looking his way when she thought no one was watching. To her he was perfect, and she? She was perfectly oblivious to the other four women he was seeing on the side. I caught him one day and spilled the beans, but Holly didn't listen and she spent years with the guy. She even ended up marrying him.

Fast forward a few years and Holly is pregnant with her first daughter, still working a nine to five job. Sebastian had lost his company and Holly was their sole provider. After a year of struggling to get by and Sebastian refusing to get any job that didn't pay enough according to him, she finally ended it and found a guy she never would've fallen for when we were in college.

Things don't always go the way we plan, and we don't get what we expect, either. It just takes something or someone to wake us up. Don't throw us away because we have other ideas. Be the person who is there when we realize that we've made a mistake.

Opposites Attract

I grew up reading the most cliché romance novels I could get my hands on. Paranormal, supernatural, contemporary, fantasy, young adult, adult, you name it. A recurring element that I have noticed is that opposites attract in nearly every one of these books. This led me to do some research on the topic. Was this even real? Did this ever happen in real life?

As it turns out, there's a whole science behind it that I won't go into explaining because no one really cares about that anyway. All you need to know is that opposites attract. Sometimes women will throw their entire checklists out the window for someone who is the complete opposite of what she had in mind. Don't let the fear of being too different stop you from going after her.

Love Comes in Unexpected Ways

Now, you've heard the story about Holly, but what I didn't tell you was how she met her current husband, Leonard.

After she dumped Sebastian, Holly didn't think she was ever going to find another man, especially not since she had a baby. She had basically given up despite my and her parents' protests. She was a single mother, living in an apartment where she had to jiggle the lock to open, with no man in sight.

Holly started taking Emily, her daughter, on playdates with people from the neighborhood. She thought it would help Emily and perhaps help herself as well. Wouldn't you know, amidst the crowd of mothers and stay at home fathers, was a single father whose wife cheated on him. With Sebastian...

This unexpected turn of events allowed them to bond, and they were inseparable. After the ugly divorce, Leonard and Holly just hit it off. Their kids became best friends and as it turned out, their fathers were college roommates.

Things happen unexpectedly, and it's a beautiful thing. Nothing and no one can predict these things. They just happen.

Leonard had no interest in business but instead focused on photography. He wasn't overly handsome, but he had a sort of attitude and confidence to him that made him more attractive than Sebastian ever was. He was the sort of man Holly overlooked for her entire life and in the end, they just happened to fall in love in the most awkward and unexpected situation.

Chapter 5: Remember What You Are Looking For, Too

Settling can be as terrible as changing your entire persona for a woman. No one should be forced to settle for a relationship or a woman. Sometimes we get so blinded by what other people want that we forget what we want entirely and that, my friends, leads to settling for someone you don't even like. Always keep your own checklist in mind when you are looking for a woman or trying to keep the one you already have. Ask yourself whether this woman is worth spending your time and effort on. Will she help you improve yourself or will she try to change you? Will you be in a relationship with her parents, or her?

Women like a man who knows what he wants and goes out and gets it. They like a man who can take a stand for what he believes in and isn't afraid to admit that he likes what he does. You shouldn't be ashamed of the person you are. Your likes and dislikes make you who you are. Sure, all people deserve a chance to prove themselves, but don't settle just because you've been together for a while, or perhaps you feel like no other woman will want you. Maybe you feel bad because you think no man will want her, either. In South Africa, they have a saying "elke pot het sy deksel" which directly translates to "every pot has a lid." The moment you or your partner has to settle, you are not each other's lids. Just like women have checklists, men have them too, and it's unfair for women to get what they want and men don't. You're worth more than settling for a woman. Women want to know that they are what you are looking for, and you will get that woman. But don't play with the one you have and drag her along, telling her that she is your lid just because you tick her boxes. A healthy relationship is about both of your boxes being ticked and both of you being happy. Above everything, women don't want to get played and lied to. We want honesty. Don't waste our time if you know we're not your lid. Remember what you want in a woman from the very start and don't forget it unless someone knocks you from your feet in that unexpected scenario.

You guessed it, another story is on its way.

When I was 17, I met Ben for the first time. He transferred from a different state and I was his designated guide through the school because we shared nearly every class. It was crazy, but at the time, I had never even kissed a boy outside of truth or dare. No boy really looked at me because I was the weird kid reading Jane Austen in the back of the class. But somehow, Ben saw me and we started dating in no time. It lasted well into college, but I knew that Ben was not my lid. He was not my prince. But for some reason, I stayed with him. Why? Because I knew that I ticked all of his boxes and I thought that I was never going to get anyone like that again. I didn't think anyone was going to want me the same way he did. Was I ever going to find another man who liked my frizzy hair and Star Wars obsession? I didn't think so, and so I settled for him, even though he was shorter than me and had the strange habit of snorting his words when he thought he was being particularly funny. It put me off, but I wanted to have a boyfriend so badly that I stuck by him.

I realized that it was unfair that I secretly hated the guy and pretended to love him. It was cruel for both of us and I knew that I had made a mistake. I didn't want to be that girl who needed a guy to feel good about herself. I knew that it wasn't an attractive trait because if a man had to do that, it would've put me off entirely.

So I broke up with him, ugly crying the entire time. I wasn't sure if it was because I thought this was the last boyfriend I was ever going to have, or if it was because he was crying. The truth is that after Ben, I kind of had a little more confidence and I taught myself to think differently. If one man could like me, there was bound to be at least one other man that could love me. I didn't have to settle. It wasn't fair to that little girl who dreamed about her prince. It wasn't fair to my future, my hopes, or my dreams.

If I haven't convinced you yet, here are some reasons why settling is a bad thing.

- You will never stop comparing her to other women

No person wants to constantly be compared to other people, especially not ones who, in some opinions, are better looking, funnier, or more perfect than they are. You will never stop comparing her to someone who actually matches your checklist and if that isn't enough to stop you, then put yourself in her shoes. If she stops and stares at every handsome man walking by, swooning and making up fantasies with them instead of you, how would that make you feel? Pretty bad, right? Don't do to others what you don't want done to yourself. Women want to know that they are the only person you have eyes for.

- Everything she does will annoy and bother you

If the two of you aren't really compatible, chances are that everything she does and says will annoy you more than anything. All of her annoying habits will be so much more prominent. If someone has annoying habits before you start dating, they're not going to disappear with time and you are not going to get used to it. It's not going to blow over and you will end up a grumpy, agitated mess because you've put yourself in a corner with a woman you never really found attractive. Settling for her isn't going to change the way you think about things or take away the things that irritate you.

- It causes a lopsided relationship

It's only natural for a person to want in return exactly what they put in. If you are settling for someone, there is no way that you will be able to give back the love and dedication that she is putting into the relationship. It will make her think that something is wrong with her and that's not what anyone wants, either. You won't be able to give any of it back because you do not feel the same way she does. You might even come to hate her because you had to settle for her and you are not getting what you want.

- You're missing out on the woman that could have been your lid

Along with "elke pot het sy deksel" there's another saying in South Africa that fits this situation perfectly. "Deur te rek vir die sterre trap jy op die blomme by jou voete," which means that by reaching for the stars, you are stepping on the flowers by your feet. Don't miss something amazing by settling for something else. You are keeping her from the person she is meant to be with, thinking that you are the one, and you are keeping yourself from the person you are supposed to be with as well.

- You'll put up with more that you should

When you are settling for someone, chances are that you will put up with more than you necessarily should because you are feeling guilty. You shouldn't have to put up with habits that drive you mad. That's not how things are supposed to be in a relationship. You will take punch after punch she hands out because you feel like you deserve it. The entire relationship will basically be you trying to make up for something you can't help.

The other alternative is that you are putting up with more than you should because you are afraid of letting go of her. Just because you don't want to be alone doesn't mean you should ignore bad or annoying things your partner does in fear of losing the relationship.

- You won't want to introduce her to your family

In my case, I dreaded introducing Ben to my family. Why? Because I knew that my parents were going to talk about him when we left, they were going to ask me about him, and I didn't want to speak about him more than necessary. I also didn't want anyone to get too attached to him because, in some way, I knew that we were never going to end up together. I didn't want him to invade my personal life either, because that meant he was becoming more a part of my life than I wanted him to.

- The sex suffers

Let's face it, if you are not attracted to a person, the sex is going to suffer. Every relationship needs sex. It's a critical part of any relationship. Whether you decided to wait until after marriage or not, sex is important. If you can't perform in bed, either she will feel as if you don't want her – which you don't – or you will become so self-conscious that you won't want to have a go at it any more than necessary.

Chapter 6: Tips & Tricks

Men think women are these complicated beings that are completely untamed, unpredictable, and crazy. Yes, men think women are crazy, but why is that? Why do they think we have some mental issues? It's because they don't understand us and the reason for that is that men think like men. You don't have the right sort of mindset to think like a woman and even grasp what goes on in our heads. So stop with your 'women are so complicated' nonsense and listen up.

The reason we act the way we do is because we think with our emotions. Men tend to hide their feelings and hide behind 'logic'. Women don't do that. We act the way our emotions tell us to. We embrace our emotions, and it's time for you as a man to embrace that too if you intend to understand the mindset of a woman.

Here are some tips and tricks on the topic.

- Every person is different

Every single person is different. Men think differently from women and every woman thinks differently. But let's focus on one thing at a time. Men and women process information differently. Just like you don't think you can understand us, women have trouble understanding men, too. This is just something we have to accept.

Now, women think differently, too. Naturally, each individual has their own thought process. Some women will talk about their feelings, and others won't even look at you. It's just the way it is. The best thing to do is not to compare women to each other. You won't be able to read one woman because you have experience with another. You have to learn the ways of the woman that you are with and handle things accordingly.

- We don't compartmentalize

Something you have to understand is that women can't shut off like men can. It sometimes astonishes me that Luke can just shut off from work as soon as he steps foot into the house, whereas I lie awake at night worrying about some meeting or another. It actually infuriates me. He doesn't understand that I worry about these things. He doesn't understand that I am stressed because of work when I am at home. So here is my advice.

Ask her about what's bothering her and listen. If she seems annoyed or agitated, it might not be because of you, so don't make the assumption that it is.

- Read our body language

As I have said, some women might tell you what's up, while others won't. But one consistent thing is our body language. That's right, we want you to figure it all out on your own. We would rather do a physical action such and pace or scowl than actually say anything about it.

- Ask

The best way to find out what's wrong is to ask. Ak her how she feels. She will tell you and it will give you a deeper understanding of what is going on in her head.

- Listen

Another thing that infuriates me is when Luke asks me how I am feeling and he instantly comes up with a solution. It's as if he doesn't listen at all. Women want to know that you are listening to them and understanding what they are going through without you having to solve her problems for her. Solving the problem comes later but until then, just shut up, listen, and comfort.

- The past is in the past, but sometimes we can't help ourselves

You know when you have a toothache and you just can't help but wiggle the tooth? That's how it is when we are angry and we bring up the past. We don't mean to. We really don't, because we know that it is unreasonable. We've had this argument before and we don't want to repeat it. But the memory does resurface every now and again and it bothers us beyond compare. Don't take it too personally when your woman brings up a mess from the past. It's most likely because she is making a connection between it and the present problem.

- Patience

Learning exactly how we think is going to take time, so be patient. Don't try to rush it because you will end up with a bigger mess than what you started with.

- It'll all pass

The most important thing to remember is that it will all blow over soon enough. Yes, we can stay angry for days at a time and hold grudges for a very long time, but it will all pass eventually. We can't stay angry or sad forever, and understand that there might be more going on in our lives than you might think.

- Don't blame hormones

'It's that time of the month' is not the reason for our feelings and outbursts. Don't blame the hormones when you've messed up because that's just going to make things worse. Sure, some women are prone to being a little more emotional than others, but don't blame hormones for every single thing.

- Consider how much she works

When stress levels are high, so are annoyance levels. Anything and everything can set us off and we can't help it. When she does get angry at something, consider how much time she spends at work or looking after the kids while still juggling everything else on top of it. That might just be the cause of her stress. Don't get angry because of a sudden outburst. All she needs is some rest. Women tend to get very grumpy when they're stressed and sleep deprived

- Put yourself in her shoes

For one moment, think of yourself as a woman and think with your emotions instead of your head. Consider everything that has happened that day in detail in the car, scrutinizing every single thing that could have been and could've gone wrong. Think with your emotions when you contemplate your position in life and looking out at the future. In that moment, what do you see? How do you feel?

- Do some research

Doing some research is a great method for putting yourself in our shoes. Not only do you get to learn about the things going on in our heads, but you also have the opportunity to learn about other methods.

Chapter 7: What do Women Want?

Right, after all that is said and done, I have come up with a list of things the majority of women find attractive and I've divided it into three parts: physical, personality, and relationship. In each of these parts, I will explain why we find each of these things attractive and maybe give you a few tips and tricks to master most of them in your own way.

Relationship

The whole idea about this book is to have a relationship, isn't it? Now here are some examples of what women want in a relationship, or a list of things that we are looking for before we fully commit to someone. These are the things we want men to do in the relationship. This being said, we don't always know what men want, and it's important to talk to each other about these things.

Not everything may be listed, or perhaps I listed too many. Every person is different, but I can give you a guideline of sorts.

Support

Support is one of the most important parts of a relationship and it's what every woman wants. It's what we all look for. In a world where everyone tells us that we can't do what we want to, whether it's job-wise, hobby-wise, or just lifestyle-wise, we need support just as much as you do. Support, like all things in a relationship, goes both ways, and although some men might think that they are the only ones that need support, women do, too. It doesn't matter what the context is. Support that woman of yours. It's in our nature to care for others, to support whoever comes our way. We're just programmed that way. But, we desire that support as well.

Respect

Respect; a seven letter word that many men are incapable of giving to women. Cat calls and inappropriate comments will win you no favors with the ladies. It's disrespectful, and quite frankly, no woman appreciates that sort of thing. We long for the days where we can walk on the sidewalk without constant whistles or vulgar remarks. Of course, not all men are like this, thank the heavens, but it would be appreciated if more men could show us the same sort of courtesy. Women want respect in general life, the workplace, and even more so in her relationship. A man who can respect a woman is a scarce thing and when we find one of those rare beings, we tend to hold on to them with all we've got. Show a little respect for a woman and her wishes and you might just win her respect and maybe, just maybe, her heart.

Stability

Whether it's emotionally, financially, or stability within the relationship itself, a woman wants all three of those things. Thousands of years ago when the survival of the human race depended on hunting with handmade spears and picking berries from bushes, women still had a sort of instinct that drew them to the strongest and most stable warrior in the clan. Why? Because it's safe. Because she knew that she was going to be safe and looked after. Much like our ancestors, women are still drawn to that sort of stability. I'm not saying you have to be a CEO, but if you have a proper, stable job, a woman will be drawn to it without even knowing it. They also want a man that's emotionally stable. One that won't have outbursts and temper tantrums. That's not hot, guys. No woman likes a man who can't control his emotions.

And lastly, they want stability in the relationship. They want it solid and don't care for having to question it. They want to know that it will be consistent and strong.

Interest

In my marriage, I struggle with this a lot. Luke is a great man. He's everything I want and need. But keeping his interest is like playing chess with a wall. He's constantly aloof and seems as if he just doesn't care enough to be interested. I know that he loves me as much as I love him, but it wouldn't hurt him to take an interest in me or the things I do.

Women want to feel as if their partner can't get enough of them; as if they are so interested that there is nothing that bores them or takes their mind off them. Show interest in them but don't interview them. There's a thin line you'll have to keep. A woman doesn't want to work for your attention, but she also doesn't want to work *for* you. Skip the interview and ask her about her childhood. Trust me, this isn't like changing your entire person to match her, it's just a state of mind you have to get in.

Equality

Forget feminism and all those controversial things for a moment and think about treating your woman as an equal. It's all we've ever wanted. Don't make decisions that affect both of you without her. She has just as much say as you do in this relationship, so show her that you know this and respect it. A woman doesn't want to feel as if you think you are better than her in any way, shape, or form. She wants to know that you are equals and have equal say in the relationship.

Acceptance

When I was a teenager, I dated a guy who I thought was the perfect match. He had a band called 'The Garage Skunks' and did bad Bon Jovi covers. As a teenage girl, I didn't care how bad they were; I was dating a guitarist! But he had this horrible tendency to mock my taste in music and style. On more than one occasion, he told me to wear more makeup and try wearing more black and leather. I told him where he could shove his guitar and never spoke to him again.

The point of this story is to explain why acceptance is important. No one should try to change anyone. This is basically telling a person, "Change your haircut and maybe then I'll like you." No, men, that is not how it works. If you're chasing after a woman or even dating her, you are with her because of who she is. If you are trying to change her, you are not the man for her. Women want acceptance of their personalities, looks, and habits. Don't be the jerk that tries to take her person away from her.

Assertiveness

Tell her what you want. Yes, if you want a backrub, tell her you want one. Not only will this make her more comfortable in sharing what she wants with you, but it will also form a bond between the two of you. Everyone is different and that means that you can't tell what exactly the other person wants without them telling you. People want different things and a woman doesn't want a relationship where she has to constantly guess what she has to do or say to make you happy. Bite the bullet and tell her you want a backrub. Not only will you get that massage, but you will also have a very happy woman. A man who isn't afraid of telling a woman what he wants is a keeper.

Romance

I remember when I was a child, my dad used to plan an entire day of cute things for Valentine's Day. I'm talking chocolate pancakes for breakfast in bed with strawberries and coffee, rose petals in the bathtub, a candle-lit dinner served by my brother Andrew and I (he used to pay us by giving us a candy bar). That is the sort of romance a woman wants. She wants to feel loved. She wants to feel appreciated and cared for. Women in general are suckers for romance, so don't be afraid to whip out a bouquet of flowers unexpectedly or flirt every so often. Woo her like you used to before you were together. Don't let the romance die down just because you have her in your clutches. The entire point of a relationship is to be romantically involved. Really men, it's in the phrase itself.

Protectiveness

There's a difference between possessiveness and protectiveness, so be careful on what side of the line you are walking. Women want to feel safe with a man. They want to know that nothing will hurt them if you had any say in it. They want to know that a man will walk the extra mile to protect them from harm. This isn't merely with other people. They don't want to be defensive around their men. My mom always said that she can handle anything as long as my dad's at her side. She said that she knew everything was going to be okay because she knew that my father would protect her and make things okay again. Let's face the facts; women are weaker than men. We don't have the same physical strength or speed by nature and our emotions are all over the place. Having a man around that we don't have to be defensive around is a big turn on, in my opinion.

Chemistry

Women want to have chemistry with their men. You need to have things to talk about, after all, and there should be a spark that makes her tummy tingle. Women want to feel energized when they talk to a man and they want to know that the man feels the same way. Women want someone to have a deep connection with in order to build a strong relationship. We don't want it to be forced from either side of the relationship. A relationship isn't only about sex. It's about the mental and social connection you have, too. Women want a relationship, not a sex buddy.

Love

Above all else, women want love in a relationship. Not the sort of love that you feel for a puppy or a brother, but the love than will make her world seem brighter and more positive. Women want the sort of passionate and intense love that you read about in books or see in movies. They want the love that makes them grin every time they think about you. It's been our dream since childhood, so don't take that away from us. If you can't give us that love, we don't want it. We want 100% or nothing.

Personality

Contrary to popular belief, women do not need macho, masculine men and you don't have to constantly try and prove that. What we want is in the personality as well. It doesn't matter if you tick all of the physical things women find attractive. If you don't have one or more of these following personality traits, chances are that you won't last long with the woman you have. Some of these things should be a given. A person has to be loyal and trustworthy. Without that, there is no relationship. Still, we live in a world where these things have to be sought after. It doesn't just come with any man.

Here is a list of the most common personality traits we look for and why.

Independence

Independence is a thing many men tend to overlook when they think about what a woman wants in a man. It's in our nature to look for a man that can stand on his own two feet and doesn't need anyone's help paying his bills or making up his own mind. Independence is also the act of being able to partake in your own hobbies and interests without dragging her along every single time. She has her own hobbies as well and it's in both of your best interests if you respect each other's interests and partake in your own hobbies. Don't be clingy. Do your thing.

Intelligence

My grandfather used to say, "If a man can learn when to keep his mouth shut, even a fool will seem intelligent." Women love men who know what there are talking about. There's nothing as terrible as going on a date with a man that can only speak about football and weightlifting. That doesn't make a person intelligent. But as my grandfather said, keep your mouth shut when the woman is speaking about something you do not know about and soak it in. Don't try to impress her, because chances are that you will look like an idiot if you confuse a jacket with a coat. Women want men intelligent enough to talk about their interests and teach them new things, while having the wits to know when to shut up and learn something new from them.

Leadership

Women love a man who can take the lead and give guidance without taking over control entirely. There is a difference between a leader and a dictator, and women don't want the latter, so be very careful when you are walking the line. Women like a man who can be a good role model and give advice without being judgmental or rude. Someone who can share his knowledge with other people without being a know-it-all is very attractive.

Good communication skills

A man with good communication skills is a good man to have around. When my relationship with Luke was just starting out, I was the shy one that didn't want to take back a shirt that was too small and he was the one who organized everything and made sure I did actually take the shirt back and not waste my money. He has taught me a lot over the years about communicating, and I will be eternally grateful for it. Women like men who can help them communicate better and teach them how to be more social.

Selflessness

There's just something about a man that cares more about others than himself that makes a woman so happy and melts her heart. Women look for men that openly display selflessness, because then they know that their relationship won't be one sided. No one wants to be in a relationship with a selfish person, and what's more opposite than a man who helps out at charities or feeds the homeless? It's wonderful to see people, not only men, but people in general perform such selfless acts. A woman won't look past your good deeds, because that is exactly what she wants in a man

Manners

Manners maketh man. I love a man who can greet properly without having a stinky attitude. Women love it when a man opens their door for them or lets them walk first into a restaurant. Manners can vary from etiquette to chivalry, all of which women eat up like chocolates. We love a man who isn't afraid to pull her chair out or wait to eat until her plate of food has arrived as well. Women are also fragile beings, and being polite and nice to them can make them relax instantly.

Family orientated

Whether you are close to your parents or want a big happy family, most women love a man who is family orientated. It says a lot about a man who loves and respects his mother, who looks up to his father and enjoys his company. A man who loves his family is a good man to have, my mother always said, and that is exactly what a lot of women look for. We want a man that isn't afraid of kissing his mother when saying goodbye or talking about children he might one day like to have. Even a father who enjoys spending time with his kid is a big plus point.

Handy

It's no secret that women aren't really good at fixing things. Not all women, anyway. Women want a man who can fix things when they are broken instead of calling a repair service. We like to watch a man do woodworking or paint the living room. Not to mention it is a totally sexy activity. Haven't you ever wondered why there are so many romance novels about a woman falling in love with the man fixing up her home for her? It's because women love knowing that there is someone who can fix, build, and keep things in order.

Understanding

I wasn't sure what to title this because it has many layers to it. Women want a man who is understanding and comforting. We want a man to understand that we are working hard and trying to build a future for ourselves. We want a man to understand that a certain time of the month we might eat more chocolates than usual. Men who don't understand how normal periods work make women really uncomfortable. They want a man who understands and offers to run her a nice, hot bath or rub her feet.

Passion

There's nothing as entertaining as watching someone who's passionate about something talk. Women love watching men explain their hobbies and likes. We enjoy seeing the childlike giddiness when you talk.

On my first date with Luke, he took me to a little Italian place that only lasted a month after opening. I asked him about his interests and his eyes lit up. I watched, chin on my hand, as he went on and on about his travels and the different sorts of cuisines he's tried in different countries. Although he's a crypto currency investor, he has a passion for cooking and eating. I've never seen a man eat like he does. It doesn't matter what you're passionate about, don't be afraid to share it. We love a man who can be passionate and excited about small things. It also gives us an idea of how passionate you are in other areas, if you know what I mean.

Good with words

Personally, I love a man who can speak well in good, educated English. Men who can use big words and actually know that they mean are very attractive and very rare. If you want to swoop a woman off her feet, don't use any of the new aged rubbish slang, and instead speak nice and pure English. It lets a woman know that you are educated and intelligent, which is something all women want in a man. We love it when a man can seduce us with words.

Sense of humor

The best way to a woman's heart is to make her laugh. A natural sense of humor is hard to come by, and one that matches ours is even better. Having a relationship where you have to walk on eggshells because you are too afraid to make the joke someone might find offensive is a terrible life to live. You have to be able to make a joke and take one. Make your woman laugh and you will have a lot of points in your favor.

Sense of responsibility

Along with independence, responsibility is a must. A woman wants a man that can take responsibility and man up. I find that a man who has responsibilities like bills and a job is far more attractive than a spoiled rich guy sponging off his parents' fortune.

Adventurous

Sure, a man who knows his way around a jungle is sexy, but that's not what I mean by adventurous. I'm talking adventurous in the relationship. Try new things, take the next step, do different things together. Women want men to take the initiative and initiate an adventure. They want you to take their hand, look them in the eyes, and tell them that you want to try something new. The special part is that you want to experience it with them. That is why women go for men with adventurous souls; men that are not afraid of trying something new and exciting.

Confidence

One of the most appealing things to a woman is a confident man. We want someone who is confident in what he does, a man that believes in himself, his work, and knows exactly what he wants. The most off-putting thing is constantly having to reassure someone about their worth. It's tiring to say the least. It will happen. Of course it will, men aren't superhumans, and naturally you will need some reassurance every now and again. But a confident man doesn't need others to tell him how much he's worth or what he has to offer. When a man is comfortable in his own skin, it will automatically make a woman more comfortable as well. Confidence is a great thing to have, regardless of what women want in a man.

Loyalty

This shouldn't even be on the list, to be perfectly honest. It's a given. Once you are with a person, you are supposed to be loyal. Loyalty isn't something that has to be earned, it's a trait everyone is supposed to have. But in today's society, it isn't given out so freely anymore, and that is why women value that so much in a partner.

Integrity

Morals, men, morals. Women desire a man with honor and strong moral principles. This mirrors your integrity involving your relationship.

Compassion

Compassion and empathy attract women like moths to a flame. Women want someone they can open up to and find comfort in. We want someone who can see our point of view and understand our hopes, fears, and dreams. We find interest in a man who shows concern and wants to care for others.

Emotional availability

You know that feeling when you are talking to someone and you have their undivided attention? That feeling when it's just you and that person with no one left around you? That's what women want, too. Someone who listens without any distractions and responds with enthusiasm. We want a man that we can talk to and share our feelings with. We want a man that can understand where we are coming from and share his own feelings as well. Some men have this idea in their heads that showing emotion makes them less manly, but it doesn't. Not sharing any feelings or emotions merely makes a man seem aloof and uninterested.

Manly

Women want a strong and manly man. It's the way that we are wired and that will never change. A man that we can feel safe around and know that, if something bad were to happen, a woman would be safe. My father is the sort of man that rarely shows that he is in pain because he believes that it makes him manly. He'd rather carry things alone and tear some muscles than ask a woman to help because it's a man's job to do the heavy lifting. Perhaps I just learned that from my father and that was what I looked for in a man.

Someone who can teach her new things

Women love a man who can teach her a new skill or two and doesn't get angry at her when she doesn't get it right the first time around. We want to learn new things and get better at what we already know. We want a patient man who is willing to teach us, no matter how long it takes. Honestly, that is one of the most attractive things a man can do; just have patience with us. No one gets something done the first time around, so just keep that in mind. Patience is always a good thing and when you pair that with something new, it's a good combination.

Ambition

What is ambition? You might stop and tell me that it's a mission you set for yourself. You might say that it's a dream. Me? I say it's a challenge you set for yourself. Women don't want a man that's comfortable in one position. It's extremely attractive if a man wants to be more than he already is. Set some goals for yourself and don't be afraid to share them with her. We like hearing about them.

Animal lover

The two best things in the world are ice scream and puppies. Now, when we can't get our hands on ice cream, the next best thing is a puppy. A man who has a soft spot for animals instantly climbs to the very top of our little books.

Good cook

I've mentioned that Luke is a foodie. What I didn't say is that Luke is the best cook I have ever known. After the first meal he cooked for me, I knew I loved him. Well, perhaps I knew I loved him the moment I watched him cook, I just realized it when I finished my second plate of food. There are a lot of hobbies women find attractive, such as woodwork and boxing, but let me tell you, a good cook? Take a cooking class or two. You'll thank me later.

Artistic

Oh, the artistic soul, what a wonderful thing that is. I have first-hand experience with artistic men and let me tell you, it's a journey and I don't regret falling for one. Luke has always loved art and claimed the spare bedroom as his very own art studio. He's not very good and he knows it but that doesn't mean that he doesn't love painting any less. Sometimes I'd just stand in the door and watch him lose himself in his art. It's a beautiful thing to see – a man who can appreciate art. As soon as a man can look at a woman the same way he looks at art, she'll know he's the one. Women love a man who can appreciate any form of art. Music, painting, literature, theater... Anything he can lose his heart in. Or maybe it's just me who has always wanted that in a man. Still, I felt it very appropriate to add this to the list.

Sober thinker

Women are impulsive and it can lead to a lot of damage in a relationship. What we need is someone who thinks with a clear mind and doesn't let his emotions dictate what he does or says. In the moment, when an argument gets so heated that a person could boil water in the tension, you need someone who is steady and level-headed. I've found that a level-headed man is much more desirable than an impulsive one. Sometimes it's better to let us cool off before matching our impulsive behavior. We don't always mean what we say but whenever you say something to us we will remember it until the day we die. Think of the future instead of the present argument is all I'm saying.

Physical

No one can do anything about their appearance, but I can name a few things that might boost your confidence a little if you are in possession of any of these features that you might not know women adore.

Good sense of style

Men, I'll let you in on a little secret; women absolutely love a man who can dress to impress. Good style is probably one of the sexiest things a man can have. There's a reason why the man in the suit usually gets the girl instead of a man in cargo shorts with socks and sandals. It doesn't matter what you look like or what body type you have. If you are wearing clothes that fit you and match your shoes, a woman is sure to swoon.

Good teeth

There's something about a man with pearly whites that gets women swooning. Good, well looked after teeth are very attractive and can be a major turn on for women.

Dad bod

In my personal experience, I've found that men with a little extra meat are more attractive than a man with a perfectly toned, bodybuilder body. Why? Because that means we don't have to constantly worry about losing those extra couple of pounds to stay "worthy" of their presence. As soon as a man has a better body than a woman, we instantly try to look out for what we eat and get self-conscious about the little spring rolls around our bellies whenever they take their shirts off. Sure, it's hot, but that doesn't mean we want that. A dad bod, in my opinion, is much more attractive when I am looking for a relationship than a man with a six pack.

However, if you do have an actor's body, don't fret! It's still sexy; just be sure to tell your woman that she doesn't need to feel the way she does around you. You shouldn't worry about her body type. If she's happy, so should you be and I wish more men with sculpted abs would just stop women from starving themselves to keep up.

Veiny forearms

Oh, honey, let me tell you something. Veiny forearms can make any woman swoon. I'm not sure what it is about it that makes us go crazy but I can assure you that those veins you might not be comfortable with can score you some major points with the fairer sex. It also represents good health and an indication that a man in possession of veiny forearms is strong.

Freckles

Freckles are the cutest things when they're on a girl, but on a man? Many women prefer freckles over clear skin. Something you might think of as an imperfection is the same thing that attracts women to you. Freckles are on a lot more checklists than you might think. Take it from a woman who has it on her own checklist.

Fluff

Sure, a perfectly smooth body is sexy in a sort of ethereal way, but ladies love a little to a lot of fluff. Body hair is a stereotypical sign of manliness and women want a man, not a waxing buddy to go to the salon with. Don't be afraid to show off those chest hairs.

Facial hair

If it wasn't a must, it would've just been called an 'ache'. Yes men, we love facial hair. Whether you have a full beard or some stubble, chances are that your woman loves that. As long as it's well looked after and groomed, it's just like body hair, to be honest. It makes you look more manly and perhaps a little mysterious. A little bit of brutish good looks has never hurt anyone. I constantly beg Luke not to shave his beard because it makes him too attractive for words. When in doubt, grow a beard.

Tattoos

This might not be for everyone. In fact, it might not be for most. But there is a handful of women, (me included) who absolutely adore tattoos. It's like looking at paintings that are on a body and we love tracing them with our fingers and hearing the stories behind them. Don't feel as if you have to hide them around people. Sure, some parents might not approve, but they aren't the ones who have to live with it for the rest of their lives. Tattoos give men that bad boy feel and women love that.

Full lips

Women love lips they can be jealous of. Why? Well, there's a lot more to kiss, obviously. Not to mention the way those lips look accompanied with a smile, smirk, or smolder. It's enough to make any woman swoon.

Scars

There's just something about scars on a man that screams "I've been places and I have these scars to prove it." It's rugged, it's masculine, and it makes you look like a total bad boy. We all know women can't resist a bad boy with a softer side. If you have scars, the former is already taken care of. Pair it with a love of puppies and we have a perfect man on our hands.

Grey hair

My brother found his first grey hair before he turned 21. Of course, as any person would, he freaked out and plucked it before anyone else saw it. By the age of 30, he had more grey hair in his beard than black and women swooned over him left right and center. This, of course, made my sister-in-law very smug because it was her man that was so hot. Grey hair usually comes from trauma, stress, or overworking yourself. It shows that you are not afraid to work, that you've experienced things and been places. It shows that you have experience in life.

Big noses

My mother always told me that men had to have bigger hands, ears, and noses than women. And, although it's not a 'must', it sure is attractive. A big nose adds character to a face and makes you look unique. Take a look at Ryan Gosling and Tom Cruise. They definitely don't have the smallest of noses but hell, they are sexy hunks of men.

Sharp jawlines

Clench those jaws, men! A man with a chiseled, defined jaw is sexy, yes, but have you tried clenching your jaw a little, too? Women find that incredibly attractive. It's the small things that women look for.

Your scent

Have you ever wondered why women love wearing men's shirts so much? Why they tend to roll over in bed and wrap themselves in your half of the covers and colonize your pillow? It's because we can't resist you scent. A man's natural scent is hot on its own, but pair that with some musky, strong cologne and she won't be able to keep her hands of you. Women love men who smell good. It's one of the most attractive things about a man. Good hygiene goes without saying, so make sure you smell nice and kick out those smelly shoes.

Glasses

Who cares if you don't have perfect vision? You get to wear specs! Rock them. Men with glasses are incredibly attractive. Attractive lensless glasses can now be purchased as accessories. This had to be for a reason, no? So, don't hide the fact that you need glasses behind contact lenses. Glasses might be an annoyance, but they sure go down well with the ladies.

Accent

As someone who has travelled the world for work, I can appreciate a good accent or two. I've noticed that some men try to hide their accents in fear of being off-putting. Stop that! Women love a good, thick accent. Personally, I am a sucker for a Russian accent. The less I can understand of what he's saying to me, the better. Every person has a certain accent they find incredibly sexy. Don't hide yours. Yours might just be the accent that she is looking for.

Sexual

Sex is about being desired, and every woman in existence wants to feel desired and wanted. We want to know that a man is hungry for our bodies and we want you to prove it every time we do the devil's tango. Just like everything else, there are many things women want in bed that men don't always realize. I am probably breaking every girl code telling you these things, but I'm willing to take one for the team. Some women don't like telling their partners what they want in bed and so the man is left trying to figure these things out on his own. Well. You're not alone. Here are some things I have learned from experience, and from research, that drive a woman wild even though she might never admit it.

Be verbal

As much as men love to hear a woman moaning their name or telling them how good something feels, women love it, too. I don't know why men find this so hard to believe, especially since an important aspect of sex for women is that they are being desired and 'enjoyed.' We love hearing you cuss under your breath when you hit a particularly sensitive nerve and we love hearing you tell us how great we feel. We also enjoy it when you tell us what you're going to do next and how. It's a big turn on.

Eye Contact

Eyes are the windows to our souls, so remind me again why men don't always make eye contact during sex? Women want that. We want you to look at as, then stare into our eyes with every orgasm. We want to see your eyes and we want it to be as intimate as possible. It makes everything feel more passionate, and you know how we feel about passion. It's a definite must.

Hands on

Women want men to touch them. Don't make us undress ourselves. Do it for us and caress our skin while you're at it. Maybe leave some kisses along the way, too. We love it when you touch and rub us during sex, too. Don't be afraid to let us know how much you love touching us. Let your hands wander and pay special attention to our intimate parts. We don't enjoy idle hands.

Kink

This isn't the first time that I'm mentioning *50 Shades of Grey*. There's a reason why the movie and the books got such a big fan base. Women love kink. Many men are afraid to try anything kinky or rough because they don't know if a woman will enjoy it. If you're not sure, ask, but if you know your woman has a wild side, get out those ties and tie her up. We love a man who can get kinky and isn't ashamed to show it. *50 Shades* was so popular because it showed us things that men never did to us and it turned us on. Take some lessons from Christian, men. You won't regret it.

Take your time

The worst thing a guy can do is rush sex. It shouldn't be just to get it over with. Sex is supposed to be an intimate act that joins people together for both pleasure and intimacy. Why would you want to rush that? Take your time on us and don't rush anything. Women want men to appreciate their bodies and explore different things. How can you do that when you are rushing to get it over with?

Make sure she finishes before you

Sex isn't just about your pleasure, it's about a woman's pleasure as well. When a man finishes, that means an end to the fun for a bit. All of your focus then goes on to other things, and many men fall asleep straight after that. Women want men to pay more attention to their needs as well. Make sure she gets her orgasm too before you finish all of the fun. Not only is it incredibly frustrating to be left high and dry – no pun intended – but it also makes us feel like you are a selfish lover.

Be spontaneous

A quickie before work has never been as hot as it is when it's spontaneous. In everyday life, we get too busy and distracted and sometimes we forget about having sex. Women don't want to be the ones who constantly initiate sex, and when you are spontaneous about it, tell her exactly how much you need her in that moment, she will be putty in your hands. We love it when you can't control your carnal desires to ravish us, so why hide it? Spontaneous sex it the best sex, in my opinion.

Get a little rough

Women love it when a man can get a little rough with her in bed. Someone who can pull our hair and give up a light spank is extremely sexy. Of course, this isn't for all women, so be careful who exactly you get rough with. Make sure she likes that sort of thing and doesn't have a past that might trigger her. Don't be afraid to ask if she would be willing to try it, though. Sometimes a woman is too shy to bring it up herself and appreciates a man who has the guts to ask such a thing.

Pay attention

Every woman is different in so many ways. Just because something worked for your ex, that doesn't mean it's going to work for your current flame. We want you to pay attention to the way our bodies react to different things you do. We want you to ask questions and listen to what we want and need. There isn't one position or method that can satisfy every single woman in the world, so ditch that idea entirely. You have to adapt to every woman differently, just like we have to adapt to men. Paying attention to our body language and listening when we speak is all we really want.

Go down on her

I know many women who say this is better than the actual dirty deed. Women love it when men go down on them and they wish men would do it more often. Of course, some women, myself included, don't enjoy it at all, so be sure you know her preferences before you eat her out. You don't have to ask her. Simply kiss a gentle trail from her neck down, and if she doesn't stop you, she's game for it. It's that much better when you know what you are doing. Women definitely want men to go down on them more often.

Foreplay

Foreplay is important to get a women hot and ready for you. Sex isn't just a physical thing for us. We need to prepare our minds and our bodies for what's about to happen. Women also take much longer than men to reach their orgasms and foreplay is a great way to get her aroused and keep her on edge, in turn making her orgasm come faster. The overall experience will be so much better, and having her aroused and turned on by you will make her take more part in the activity as well, as she will want her orgasm that much more.

Bring in some toys

Some men might find this insulting, and to be honest I don't really get why that would be. Women love it when you incorporate different and new things into your sex life. A vibrator or whatever other toy you decide to add into the mix is made to increase her pleasure, not take over for you. It's not that you are doing anything wrong. In fact, I am certain that you will be doing something incredibly right. Women love a man who can use toys on her without getting embarrassed. Also, remember that we will ask you to take control of the toy if necessary. It's impossible for you to know exactly where the vibrator has to sit for the best results, so leave the positioning to us.

Compliment her

Women want to hear what effect our body has on you. We want to know how much we turn you on, or how beautiful you think we are underneath you. We want you to shower us with compliments. Why? Because it makes us feel wanted and appreciated, which is exactly what every person wants in life. I've spoken to a bunch of women on the topic, and every single one of them said they wished their men would compliment them more during sex. One sentence is enough to send them over the edge of orgasm.

Chapter 8: What don't Women Want?

As many things as there are that we do want, there are also a wealth of things we don't want. I haven't listed everything that women want, because that would require an entire series on its own, but I can tell you some things they don't want as well, which will give you a much better idea of what we are after. There are just as many things we don't want as what we do want, so get out your notebook and make lists. Perhaps you need to take these into consideration and improve on them a little if you are in possession of any of these traits.

Relationship

Some relationships are just toxic, and anything in this category has the potential to make the relationship bad for both of you. Most of these things are general things that anyone in a relationship finds annoying and off-putting. These are only a few things that women don't want in a relationship and avoid at all cost. Usually, when we see the first red flag, we'll leave because any and all of the following things in a relationship are no other color than red. Sometimes it's easy to misinterpret other traits as one of these, so be sure to be very careful. It might just put a woman off entirely.

Feeling insecure

When a man constantly insults or mocks a woman, chances are that she will start feeling insecure about everything she does or says, and even what she looks like. We don't want to feel insecure in our own homes, so don't make us feel that way. If you don't have constructive criticism, keep quiet.

Assumptions

Assuming you know someone can lead you down a dangerous path. Women don't want a man to assume that, just because she came home later than usual, suddenly she's seeing someone else. Also, assuming that she is happy when you do certain things is also a big no-no. Read her body language and if you can't, ask. We'll appreciate you asking us much more than you just assuming things about us that are completely bogus. Women want a man who doesn't just assume things. We want a man who is sure of his facts before he confronts us.

Hearing and not listening

You know that feeling when you are talking to someone, but you know that they are not listening to you? They just bob their heads and pretend to agree with everything that you are saying just to keep the peace? Women hate that as much as you do, so don't even think about doing that. It's frustrating and it makes us feel as if you never listen to anything we say because you aren't interested in our thoughts and opinions. Personally, that's a big insult and it's not fair toward any person to do that. Rather, end the conversation when you are not interested in hearing any more.

Disrespect

Any woman with self-respect will never tolerate a man who disrespects or belittles her. We want to be treated well. Some women struggle with their self-worth, and they don't need a man disrespecting them to make them feel even worse about themselves. We need men who can compliment and respect us, men who can help us up and teach us how to respect ourselves when we are in the darkest of holes. Most women look for a man with enough respect for himself to respect the women around him, too.

Comments about her weight

Honestly, why any man would think commenting on a woman's weight is a good thing, I will never understand. It's insulting and we are already so self-conscious about our image that we don't need a man to comment on it, too. With all the skinny and fit actresses and models, we already feel inferior. Don't comment on the few pounds she picked up over the Christmas holiday. Her weight has nothing to do with you anyway. It wouldn't be the first time a woman left a man because he called her fat. Women want to be complimented, not broken down.

Controlling her

We aren't remote control cars, so stop treating us as such. We want to be independent and live our own lives. You are a part of her life and she is allowing you in. Her life doesn't become yours the instant you two start dating. We don't want a man to tell us what to wear and we sure don't want to ask permission when we want to go out with our friends. If you think you have a say in anything, you have a surprise coming your way, honey. We don't want to date a puppet master.

Cheating

I think perhaps cheating is the worst thing you can do in a relationship. Not only is it morally out of the question, but it is also an insult to the woman that you are dating. If you are dating, women want to know that you are her boyfriend and no one else's. We don't like sharing and if you are having issues with the relationship, whether it's on a metal or physical level, rather be honest with her about it than go around with another woman. Things can be sorted out more often than not, and it doesn't have to go as far as cheating. There is no excuse for that and any woman who respects herself will not stand for it.

Jealousy

There's a difference between possessiveness and jealousy. There is a thin line between the two, so be careful on which side of that line you are standing. Jealousy is a sign of insecurity, and we don't have the time to reassure you every second of every day that our guy friends are just friends. Or no, the waiter was just being nice. We want a confident man who can trust us around our friends even if they are not women.

Neglect

Women want your time and attention the same way that we are giving you ours. Women don't want a man who neglects her one day and then waltzes back into her life the next with promises of being better. We are bound to be skeptical, so just skip the neglect altogether. We are in a relationship because we want a companion, not a ghost who only appears every now and then to give us minimal amounts of attention and time. If you are that guy, she is going to get sick of the games very quickly.

Excuses

You know that story about the boy who cried wolf? That's exactly the same when it comes to excuses. Sure, sometimes things happen that we can't always help, and then they aren't really excuses, they're more like explanations. But when it becomes a constant thing in a relationship, it becomes tedious and she will get sick of it really soon. Women don't want men who constantly make excuses. If you don't want to see her, don't make excuses. Just be honest and tell her that you'd rather spend the night alone. We value honesty more than excuses.

Cancelling

It takes a lot for me to get excited for any sort of social event. I'm not a very socially active person and I am more than happy in my own little world with my family. So, in the case where I do get excited about a social event, or actually, anything that involves leaving my house, I don't want to be cancelled on at the last possible second. Don't promise a woman something and not see it through because you will end up looking at her back as she walks away from you. We want someone who we can rely on and trust.

Personality

There are too many personality traits that put us off to even count. I wouldn't say that it's just women who find these unattractive because, let's face it, most of these things are enough to put any person off. Here is a list of things in your personality you might want to work on.

Being too easy going

Throw the "happy wife, happy life" thing out of the window because that is complete and utter rubbish. Women don't like a man who just agrees with everything she says. It just infuriates her. Women want a man who can say his piece and fight for what he wants and believes in, too.

Know-it-all

I used to date a guy that drove my father mad. This man used to tell my father, an airplane enthusiast and war veteran, all about the Nazi planes and strategies. Whenever my father told him that he was wrong, the boyfriend of mine argued until he was blue in the face. He used to tell my mother about interior decorating, and lectured my brother on motorbikes. There was absolutely nothing that he didn't know. It drove me mad and eventually made me break up with him. He, of course, couldn't understand why I could do such a thing, especially since he was so intelligent. It was extremely off-putting. No woman wants a know-it-all.

Judgemental

Women don't want to feel as if they are permanently being judged. Having to worry about everything you do or say in fear of being judged is not the making of a great relationship. So what if we didn't shave all winter, did you trim your beard in the past week? We don't want to be judged by the person that is supposed to love us more than anything. If you feel the need to judge, keep your opinion to yourself because, trust me, you will either hurt her or start an argument you wish you had avoided. She might just tell you exactly what you are doing wrong, as well.

Hot-headedness

We don't want to walk on eggshells every time we communicate with our man, out of fear of set him off. Hot headedness really isn't a very attractive trait to have and I'd suggest shedding it very quickly. We don't want a man who is constantly on edge. We don't want to wait with anxiety until you finally snap and lose all your marbles, waking the neighbors up with your yelling. At the first sign that you are hot-headed or have a short temper, she will bail if she knows what's good for her because those are more often than not warning signs of a terrible relationship.

"I'm Fine"

Women are just as guilty as men when it comes to this phrase. We can clearly see when you are fine and not fine. We can tell it in the way you act, speak, and handle yourself. Don't insult us by saying that one phrase over and over again. It also makes you look as if you have a total lack of emotions and it makes any woman skeptical of you. Not only does it annoy us to no end, it also makes us trust you less.

Addictions

Any and all addictions wave red flags at us. We've seen too many dramas, too many documentaries, and have gotten too many speeches from our parents that warn us against men with addictions. Whether it's sleeping pills, alcohol, or drugs, everything is bad. There might be a few individuals that might feel it's their duty to help a man through it and show him the right way, but women tend to run away from baggage, and trust me, addiction is a lot of baggage. Women don't want to constantly worry whether or not their man is back on his pills or drugs again. It's a terrible life to live. Women don't want that for themselves and I don't blame them.

Unstable

A moody and unstable man makes any woman run for the hills. We want to be able to predict how a man will react to things we tell him and we want to know that he won't suddenly flip out and have a temper tantrum. Unstable men will also make us feel unsafe when we are under the same roof, alone and away from other people. That is not the feeling we want to have when we are with the man we love. Being moody doesn't make you brooding and mysterious, it makes you dangerous and it gets tiresome after a while.

Arrogance

Women want a man who's completely and utterly in love with them and no one else. When you are arrogant, you come across as loving yourself more than you can love anyone else. It is also a cover for insecurity, which makes this even worse. It all comes back to confidence, and that is what we really want in a man. Confidence is believing in yourself without coming across as a giant jerk, whereas arrogance makes you look like a narcissist and trust me, no woman wants to be with a narcissist. Especially when they like themselves more than they like their woman. Go on a date with yourself if you are so in love with yourself, then.

Taking things too personally

Sure, we love a man who can be sensitive and vulnerable, but as soon as you take everything too personally, it's a major turn-off. That is taking the trait that a lot of women find irresistible just a little too far. If you read into everything your partner says, she will have to think twice every time she speaks because she will be afraid of an argument or outburst. Life is fun and sometimes we make jokes that could come across as insulting when it really wasn't meant that way. Don't look into it too much.

Being overly sarcastic

I pride myself on my witty and sarcastic nature, but I know that it can sometimes get too much and I have to dial it down a notch or two. The key is knowing when to stop and when to begin. Timing is everything. It's also important to know which things you can be sarcastic about and which things to rather leave alone. It can also make a woman feel as if you are mocking her which isn't something you want to do, is it? Sarcasm isn't bad, we just don't want a man who can't have a conversation without needing to prove his wit.

Unreliable

Women want a man they can rely on. When we're stuck next to the road with a flat tire, we want to know that we can rely on our man to come help us. Unreliable men rarely get the girl because they usually tend to rely on us while we can't do the same. It's very annoying and has been etched into our brains since childhood by our parents. Reliability is one of the first things women look for in a man, and it's clear to see why. We want to know that you are going to be there for us when we need you and that you are going to come through when you said that you would.

Caring too much about what other people think

I dated a guy that was a little shorter than me and it bothered him to no end. I wasn't allowed to wear heels because he felt as if people were looking at us too much. This annoyed me so much because, not only couldn't I wear heels when I wanted to – I had to take off my heels at work and replace them with flats if I planned on going out with him that night – and it made me feel huge. As if it was my fault for being taller than him and other people's opinions bothered him. I didn't mind it. It was just one of those things. His height, despite what he tells people, was not what ended our relationship. It was his obsession with other people's opinions that I couldn't handle anymore.

Workaholics

My dad has this horrible habit of talking about work 24/7. It drives my mother and me mad and I vowed that I never wanted a man like that. The worst part is if a man is at work all the time and then when he comes home, he doesn't spend time with his partner. Instead, he spends more time with his work. We support your work and ambitions, but leave it at the office when you come home. We are with you because of *you,* not your job.

Attention hog

It's hard to be with someone who wants to be the center of attention all the time. This makes it difficult to interact with a person because your attention is bound to wander sometimes. It also causes you to be too clingy which is a turn-off all on its own. Attention hogs might get the attention of women sometimes, but it also means that we are going to get sick and tired of it eventually and then we are out of the door. We don't want men who have to be the center of attention all the time. It's tiring.

Drama

Sure, a lot of women love drama, but if we want to get it, we'll go watch the beauty community on YouTube have a go at it. We don't want drama from the men in our lives. That's not what we're looking for in a man at all. We want a stable and reliable relationship, and as soon as the curtain drops and the drama comes out, we can see the red flags from a mile away. Men who love spreading drama also have the tendency to overreact and victimize themselves. Leave the drama to the professionals, men. Women don't want to date a drama queen.

Liars

Being lied to is the most humiliating thing that could happen to a person. It's terrible, it really is. Women don't want liars because it makes us doubt everything you say. Liars are also the makings of a cheater, which makes every woman paranoid. Most liars then have the audacity to be insulted when we don't believe them when they're actually telling the truth. So just keep it real and don't lie to us and we won't lie to you.

Negativity

Negative people can have a terrible effect on our lives. I'm not saying you are never allowed to complain when the world gets you down. It happens to the best of us. Just don't let the negativity consume you entirely until you can't get out of the hole. It has a terrible effect on a relationship and that isn't the sort of person you want to spend the rest of your life with. Life is hard enough as it is and we don't need other people to rub their negativity off on us. Women don't want a man who moans and groans all the time.

Suck ups

I always hated that kid in school who used to remind the teacher of a pop quiz and announced that he did his homework while no one else did just to score some brownie points. I couldn't stand that kid and that is why it is so off-putting to have a brown-nosing boyfriend. Just be you and don't suck up to her parents or friends. That is really not something a woman wants in a man.

Bad tippers

I can totally understand if a man doesn't have a lot of money to take a woman out on fancy dates and tip the waiter like they deserve to be tipped. This might not be something men know we look out for, but we definitely do. Rather than taking her out to an expensive restaurant and giving your waiter a 1% tip, go to a cheaper place and pay the waiter what he's owed. It's a very attractive thing when a man tips and thanks the waiter properly. A stingy date is very annoying.

Bully

Many girls were subjected to bullying in school and even outside of school. I, for one, was bullied a lot.

It was just how it was. Many women share this opinion with me. Bullies are not hot. Making someone else feel like a loser just to make yourself feel better is not something a woman wants in a man. Trust me. You do not need to belittle other people just to make an impression. It's not cool, it's not nice, and it is very obnoxious. Don't fool yourself by thinking any woman wants that.

Inconsiderate

In our everyday life, we need to be considerate of people's feelings, comings and goings, and their day to day life. If you are going out with a woman and take her to a sushi bar, not even considering her allergy to fish, you are going to walk a long way home without so much as a goodnight kiss. Honest mistakes happen, but if you know for a fact that someone doesn't like a horror movie and you are inconsiderate enough to take her to watch a horror movie, you deserve the hate you're going to get from her. Take her feelings and preferences into consideration.

Loud

Those men who talk so loudly that you can't even hear yourself think just so other people can hear what they are saying, is a big "no" from me. No, I don't want to hear about the big investment you made. No, I don't care that you are going golfing with Donald Trump and no, I do not care about your brand, spanking new car that still smells new. No one cares. The worst is when a man draws too much attention to himself, especially when he is complimenting a woman or making a move. Loud people also tend to get obnoxious really quickly.

Physical

There are things that people can't change, and then there are things that they can. Everything I have listed below is something that can be improved or "fixed." These physical things are proven to put women off and as shallow as it might seem, it's true. There are things on this list that put me off as well. It's the way we function as human beings.

Things are very visual for us and if something isn't pleasing, well... Let's just say that it won't interest us at all. If you insist on fixing yourself physically, here are some things to look out for.

Fighting

I know you want to show off your masculinity somehow, but this is not the way to do it, my friend. Women don't like a fighter and they don't find it impressive when you knock a man to the ground in under five seconds. What we really want is a man who can swallow his pride and walk away like man. Real men don't have to prove anything because they have already proven what a man they really are. If you are getting attacked, it's an entirely different story, but women don't want men who pick fights.

Steroid junkie

Sure, a well-toned and muscular body is attractive, but at some point you have to realize that you are overdoing it a bit. It's all well and good until your biceps turn into pumpkins and your jeans look like tights. Good health and exercise have never been bad things, but there is a line that a person shouldn't cross. Once you go from Chris Hemsworth to Arnold Schwarzeneggar, you know that you have crossed the line. Women don't want to date a ball of muscle. It's not as attractive as you might think.

Femininity

This is a bit controversial because people don't really understand what it means when a woman says she doesn't want a feminine man. It's not a bad thing, but as soon as a man starts crying about a papercut, it puts a woman off entirely. We want a man who's tough, a man who can change the tire without complaining about his hands the entire time. We want a man's man. Sensitivity and emotional availability does not mean that you are feminine. Being a wimp in a case where women aren't makes you feminine.

Patchy facial hair

As much as we love facial hair, we prefer it being full and thick, rather than the teenage patch many men sport. That is not a beard, that is fluff. You look much better without it, trust me. In the olden days, beards were a symbol of masculinity but in the present day, it is perfectly acceptable to shave the beard off entirely. Rather hide the fact that you can't grow a beard than think you are very cool with your fluff. Women absolutely hate it when men rock the patchy fluff idea.

Bad hygiene

Have you ever stood next to a person who smells like fish and onions? It's not a lot of fun, is it? I suppose women are more obsessed with good hygiene than a lot of men and it's not a bad thing. If you know you sweat a lot, wear deodorant or at least bathe frequently. Women love the scent of a man and we love nuzzling our noses into the crook of your neck to smell you. But that is only if you have good hygiene. If you don't smell so fresh, you are not going to get into any of our good books. I can assure you of that.

Long toenails

Nails freak me out in general. Whenever we have to watch a movie where nails get ripped off, I lose it. I can't watch. The same goes for long toenails. It's gross. Just because you are a man does not mean you shouldn't take care of yourself and your body. Whenever I see an attractive man with long toenails, I lose interest entirely and I thank God for giving me a man with the same obsession with nails as I have. Long toenails put women off, point. There's also no reason for you to have them because it is most definitely not in style.

Dirty hands

Dirty hands and nails can put any woman off. I don't care if you've worked in the garden or the car, it's normal to have dirty hands after that. But when a lady goes on a date with you and she sees gunk under your nails, she is going to run for the hills. Not only is it terribly unhygienic, but it isn't very nice to look at either. A man with nice, cared for hands stands miles above a man with black fingernails and mucky hands. Women don't want to be touched by dirty hands.

Chapped lips

Everyone gets chapped lips. It's just the way of life. But that is why there is something like lip balm that we can put over it. It's the absolute worst feeling when you kiss someone and it feels as if you are kissing an alligator instead of his lips. Women have a tendency to look at men's mouths a lot when they speak, so it is always very obvious to us. Using lip balm does not make you any less of a man, and kissing you makes it that much more pleasurable for a woman when your lips are soft.

Bushy eyebrows

I get the whole strong brow thing, I do, but would it kill you to pluck your eyebrows every now and again? A man's eyebrows shouldn't be groomed to perfection like a woman's, but they shouldn't connect into one another either. A monobrow can easily make you look unattractive and despite everything I have said, women still go for attractive guys more often than less attractive guys. A monobrow can easily move you from the attractive side of the bar, to the not so attractive side. Buy some tweezers and groom those eyebrows. You'll thank me for it later.

Socks and sandals

Has this ever been in style? I don't think so, so why do some men still insist on wearing this in public? It instantly puts a woman off, trust me. If you compare socks and sandals to trainers or sneakers, which one looks better and more sophisticated? Definitely not the socks and sandals. It is a trend that has to die for the sake of humanity. Women don't go for men who wear socks and sandals and that is a fact, my friends. They never have and never will. You don't have to wear dress shoes all the time, just ditch the socks if you are so adamant about wearing sandals.

Smug grin

There's nothing as infuriating as a smug grin on someone's face. It instantly makes a person look like a jerk without them even having to open their mouth. This grin is what girls are taught to stay away from, so if you are in possession of this grin and you are wondering why women don't like you, that might be it. There's a lot that could be said about a person by the way they smile, and a smug grin is not the sort of story you want to tell a potential partner.

Pasty skin

There's just something about pasty white skin that makes a person look sickly. It's different for a woman. When she is pale it's beautiful, but as soon as a man is pale, they look ill and weak. I didn't make the rules here. When I was researching this specific point, I asked a bunch of women what they prefer: a pale man or a tanned one. All of them, and I am not exaggerating, said that they'd rather go for a tanned man than a pale one. Pale skin also insinuates that you spend a lot of time indoors, and to some it might be called laziness even though many jobs require a person to be indoors all the time. It wouldn't hurt to get a tan, though.

Man bun

I never understood why men decided that man buns were a thing. The vote is about 50/50 on this, but I felt the need to put it in this section of the book because of how much I personally hate a man bun. Especially when the sides of your head are shaved and it looks like you are wearing a toupee on a shaved head and forgot to add the sides, too. Some women, like myself, really hate this style.

Dirty hair

Oily or greasy hair can easily make you look like a slob and trust me, that is not what any woman wants to date. Make sure that your hair always smells and looks clean and fresh.

Long, thin hair

My cousin's child was unfortunate enough to have been a teenager in the early 2000's. Which meant Hot Topic vests and emo hair. Now see, Brayden is a beautiful boy, he really is. The ladies swoon whenever he walks by, but he has the thinnest hair I have ever seen on a man. You can't see it when it's short and groomed, but with the emo bangs he reminded me a lot of Gollum from *The Lord of the Rings*. The thin hair, that is. Whenever you can see onto your scalp with longer hair, it's time to cut it. I don't care if you really want long hair. Unless you want to look like a fictional character, I'd suggest cutting it all off. Women always look at hair and once they see that wreck on a head, they will walk right past you.

Sexual

If only more men would listen to what women want and don't want sexually, the world would be a much better place. I once heard a friend of mine say that if babies were determined by women's orgasms, overpopulation would never have been a problem, and it's true. These are a few things we definitely don't want in bed, and you would do well to stay away from them. Many women have cut men loose for far less than a bad sex life.

Being too quiet

Men like women to make a lot of noise during sex, right? Then why do some men try their best not to make so much as a sound? I was with a guy – the short one – who refused to make a sound. I could literally see him pulling his face in ungodly ways just so he didn't have to moan. It infuriated me. Women want to hear men as much as men want to hear women. It doesn't make you tough not to make a sound, it makes you stupid because we love it. Women want men who can moan their way through an orgasm without holding back. It gives us a little satisfaction, you know?

Bragging

Never, ever brag about how good you are in bed without proving yourself first. Women hate being told that their lives are going to be rocked when you are the most vanilla, average dude in bed. We hate being disappointed, so instead of running that risk, rather show her what you're made of before you talk about your magic wand and all the glorious things you can do with it. Not to mention the awkwardness when you don't know what to say when someone is bragging away. Women don't like braggers. Not with sex and not with anything else.

Being selfish

Sex isn't only about your pleasure. It's about both parties' pleasure. Don't be a selfish jerk and only do the things you like and then, without warning, finish before she does. I've mentioned this before and I will do so again just to get it into your head. You never finish before a lady does. Make sure she has had her fun as well before you roll over and pass out. Don't make her responsible for her own orgasms because trust me, she will dump you to find someone who is willing to make her feel as good as she makes him feel.

Going your own rhythm

When a woman tells you "yes, that's it" she doesn't mean go faster or harder. She means you should go on just like that. Women want a man who listens to her, who doesn't do his own thing when they are together. This isn't only about you, this is about her as well, and if you are going your own rhythm without taking her into consideration, you won't be spending the night at her place, that's for certain. This will deprive her of her orgasm and lead you to yours before she gets anything.

Kissing with gum

Unfortunately, I have had this happen to me on multiple occasions and every single time I end up with their gum in my mouth. I don't understand why some men find this so sexy. If you are going to make out with me, at least take the gum out of your mouth first. If you can't be mature enough to spit your gum out, then I can't be bothered to kiss you. Women don't want to chew on your pre-chewed gum, thank you very much.

Laziness

Letting her do all of the work is a complete jerk move, and if she doesn't throw you out after that first time it happens, you better make sure you don't let it happen again. Sex is supposed to be a 50/50 activity and if she has to do all of the work, she might feel as if you are using her for the sex alone. But if you put in as much effort as she does, then she'll know that it is a team effort and it will pay off for both of you in the end. Women don't want men who just lie on their backs and expect her to do all the work.

Bad breath

I have one rule about kissing other than the gum one and that is this: don't kiss me with stinky breath. I am lucky enough not to have a morning breath and neither does Luke, so we get to kiss as soon as we wake up. He also knows not to kiss me directly after we had a meal when a person can still vaguely taste the meal. Breath mints are not so hard to come by. Women hate men who kiss them with smelly breath.

No communication

You have to communicate with a woman if you intend on giving her the pleasure she deserves. She might not be outgoing enough to tell you what she likes and dislikes straight off the bat, and that is why you have to ask her how it was or what she would want to do differently next time. If she tells you, it's not your place to get upset or offended.

Everyone does things the other person doesn't like, so it's nothing to be offended about. If you are finding something not to your liking and you don't mention it, women hate it when you bring it up at a later stage or in an argument. Communication is key.

Expecting oral

Wanting a blowjob is a natural thing for a man and it's really not that strange, but there is a difference between wanting oral and expecting it. Women get annoyed by men who get angry when the woman doesn't want to give a blowjob. You have to understand that some of us just don't like doing it. There might be other things that we are game to try, but if you want to be a jerk about it, she might not even be willing to try any of the other things anymore. Oral is not something you expect, it's a gift when you get it.

Rushing foreplay

As we have learned, foreplay is the foundation of great sex. Some might even say it's the best part. Men who rush or skip this entirely rob a woman. This is the time for us to get aroused. This is the time to set the mood and turn us on. That natural lube also helps for the sex to be as comfortable and pain free as possible. Why would you want to take that away from us? Women want a man who can turn them on with his words and fingers alone. They want a man who enjoys turning them on and goes all out with foreplay.

Talking about previous lovers

Women don't want to be compared to other women sexually or in any other way. Never bring up how great your sex was with an ex because she will tell you to take your things and go back to that woman if she was so great. It's also common knowledge that you should never bring up an ex when you are in a new relationship unless she specifically asks you about them. Even then, you keep the details about your steamy sex life to yourself, you hear? You will be in big trouble otherwise

Being too aggressive

This is something most men get wrong and I am here to help. There is a difference between wild, rough sex and aggressive sex. Being too passionate can lead to aggressive and sometimes painful sex. If she is into the aggression, she will let you know and if you want to go a little rough on her, make sure that you are not taking it too far. Sex is about pleasure and not pain in normal relationships. Remember that.

Conclusion

Let's go over what we've learned, shall we?

First and foremost, nobody's perfect and everybody is different. That's the beauty of the world. We should never strive to be like someone else. That's not improvement, that's cloning, and no one wants a clone.

It's also important to know and remember who you are. Many things can be learned to improve yourself as a person. Do that instead of changing who you are entirely.

What you want is important as well. It's not merely about what women want in men, but what men want in women as well. That's a book for an entirely different day, but it's a good thing to remember. Don't compromise.

Women think differently and that's why men like to say we're so overly complicated. Men don't understand or even make the effort of understanding what goes on in our heads and all of a sudden we are these mysterious creatures that no one can figure out.

There are long lists of things women generally want in a man and looking at the lists will make any person's blood chill. However, what we want is not that unreasonable. Wanting a trustworthy, loyal man is not too much to ask for. If you make the effort to read into what we want, you'll see that it's not all superficial. Sure, a handsome man has never been ugly, but most women will go for a man with a personality that matches her list instead of a Calvin Klein model and that is the truth, my friend. Women don't only look for traits in men, but they look for certain things in a relationship as well.

In conclusion, women are not as complicated as you might think.

Moving on - If you've made it this far in the book, chances are you are still waiting for me to spill those secrets, huh? Let me give you a little backstory.

It's the 90's and I'm in my senior year. I'm wearing my usual denim dungarees and converse sneakers. I have too many braids in my hair that lead to pigtails. It was all the rage back then. I don't know how. It wasn't pretty then either. I had just gotten a new eyeshadow pallet with the metallic blue that, at the time, I thought would make my eyes pop. Now that I look back, I really did look like I had an extra eyelid with no lashes. Ah, the '90s were awesome.

I'm at a party in a clearing in the woods. Everyone's VW Beetles were parked in a row and Max's van had a stereo loud enough to give the whole party music. ABBA was playing in the background and drinks were flowing, marijuana being smoked like kids vaping nowadays. It was the final party before the real grind at school began, and Max felt it was appropriate to throw the biggest, loudest party he possibly could. Max was about as obnoxious as he sounds.

There were kids from other schools there, too. As usual, the football jocks were looking for fights with each other and the cheerleaders spoke smack about everyone else. It was just another high school party. My best friend at the time couldn't make it because of family responsibilities but she left me in charge of watching over Max, her boyfriend. He was a real Casanova and liked the ladies too much for his own good. I never knew what she saw in him until that night.

Max and I were sharing a blunt as we say in the back of his van, the door wide open so we could look at the sky, talking about the stars and what life could be possible beyond the universe that we are in, you know? Like one does. We've never really had the opportunity to talk like we did that night. He wasn't as brainless as I thought, and it might have been the devil's lettuce or the poor lighting from the bonfire, but he actually began looking a little attractive.

After contemplating the possibilities of extraterrestrials, one thing led to another and we kissed. Then the doors of the van closed and I lost my virginity in the back of my best friend's boyfriend's van… To my best friend's boyfriend.

It was a terrible thing to do and we were so young – and so high. We agreed never to bring it up again. I've never even told Luke. You are the first to learn this secret.

There's a connection with the story and this book.

Max wasn't what either I or my best friend were looking for in a man. Not even close to it. But it took a man like him for me to realize what I did and didn't want in a man. It takes a lot of experience, a lot of affairs and relationships to realize what you actually want. You can't want something you've never experienced and you can't knock it 'til you've tried it. Men are able to change our minds for the better or the worse. Just because we might have an idea of something in our heads, that doesn't mean our minds can't change for the right person.

I hope this book helped you understand us better and get a better grasp on the things we want in a man and in a relationship.

This is my first book and there is still a lot I can learn, but I am glad to share the knowledge I do have to give you a little boost of confidence, understanding, and perhaps a better idea about the mind of a woman. We're really not as complicated as men want to believe we are. We just think a little differently, that's all.

Remember, don't change but rather improve. Don't lie about who you are, but rather be honest and give the woman a chance to get to know you and maybe change her mind on a lot of things. And above all else, be confident in the person you are. It's enough to make any woman swoon.

As this is my first book, I would very much like if you could leave a review. I want to know what I can improve on, add, or remove in my books to come. It is my goal to help as many people as I possibly can with my advice, tips, and tricks. Please let me know if this was helpful.